Look Younger and More Attractive In 7 Days or Less

Beverly Paul

Copyright

Terms of Use

Any information provided in this book is through the author's interpretation. The author has done strenuous work to reassure the accuracy of this subject. If you wish you attempt any of the practices provided in this book, you are doing so with your own responsibility. The author will not be held accountable for any misinterpretations or misrepresentations of the information provided here.

All information provided is done so with every effort to represent the subject, but does not guarantee that your life will change. The author shall not be held liable for any direct or indirect damages that result from reading this book.

Contents

Copyright   2

Terms of Use   3

Introduction   5

It is All in Your Head   9

Lifestyle   13

Environment   17

Tips to Look Good – Quickly   21

Body Language Counts   25

The Attraction Factor   31

Make a Power Play   35

Quick Tips for Style and Fashion   39

Wardrobe Know How   43

Take Care of Your Skin   51

Anti-Aging   55

Quick Tips to Look Young   59

Makeup   63

Personality Traits   67

Professional Success   71

Energize Your Body   75

Sex Appeal   79

Watch Out for Stress   83

Be Positive   87

Energize Your Mind   91

Conclusion   95

Introduction

The great dilemma about life is that nobody wants to get old and yet nobody wants to die young either. As technology advances, we have been able to live longer and healthier lives than those of our ancestors. With medical breakthroughs, we are no longer as susceptible to disease and our hospitals are able to mend us when we are hurt or ill. However, aging is still something that we all do, and there is no medical procedure or pill to take to stop the march of time.

The key to staying younger has always been of interest to people. The Fountain of Youth, that tantalizing promise of youth from its waters has always eluded the grasp of those who have sought it out. Entire expeditions were launched to look for this glorious miracle and yet it was never discovered. Science has tried to come up with their own "fountain of youth". Walk into any drug store and go to the health and beauty aisle, you will find numerous lotions and creams all promising to erase wrinkles and turn back the clock.

There are pills, creams, lotions, even exercise devices all claiming to the miracle that stops aging. There is a huge market for anti-aging products and it is ever growing, despite there being no real proof that any of these work. However, people buy them, hoping. We all want to retain our youthful appearance, the glowing and smooth skin, the pep in our step, the days when we had no aches and pains.

Also on those shelves in the drug store, make up, creams, lotions and pills to change our appearance. We are also in a quest to be more attractive, to look the best that we possibly can. Both the anti-aging and the products designed to make us more attractive are playing off on the most basic of human needs, our self-esteem. Who would not want to be more attractive and younger?

These products are targeting the outside of our bodies, and some claim to work from the inside out, as is the case with the supplements. However, the keys to looking younger, feeling younger and feeling and appearing more attractive to others is not found on the shelves of your local drug store. It is already in you to have that more youthful appearance, to feel and be more attractive.

You already have the tools to help you achieve all of that and you do not need to break the bank and fill your shelves with costly products that in the end do nothing but take up space in your cabinet.

Part of the key is diet, watching what you put into your body is important, especially drugs, alcohol, smoking and overly fatty and processed foods. What we put into our bodies is very important.

Another key thing is feeling young, exercise to stay limber and keep our joints moving. You are only as old as you feel.

The main part, especially for being and feeling more attractive is mental. Our attitudes affect our mental outlook and our moods. When we feel positive, we look positive and act positive and therefore, more attractive. People are more apt to pay attention to somebody who is smiling and engaging in conversation with people rather than the person who stays in the back, watching the flood, with a scowl on their face.

We will take you through some of the basics for feeling, looking and appearing more youthful and attractive and it will not require you to buy fancy products, we will simply give you some good living tips and help you use the tools you already have.

It is All in Your Head

There is a connection between our minds and our bodies. Our automatic nervous system is controlled by our brain; and the automatic nervous system controls our automatic bodily functions like our breathing, heartbeat, digestion, and blood pressure.

Our emotions can have an effect on these automatic functions. When angry, stressed, or fearful, we breathe harder, our heat beats faster, our blood pressure raises. When we are worried or anxious we also produce more stomach acid. All of things are in response to our negative emotions and all of these bodily reactions have dangerous effects on our health long term.

Laughter triggers the release of endorphins in the brain; these relax the cardiovascular system. When we laugh, we feel good. Seems too simple; but it really is that simple.

Therefore, if negative emotions affect our health negatively, it goes to follow that positive ones affect our health in positive ways. One such benefit is the endorphins. Another is when we do not have the stressors on the body that the negative emotions have such as elevated blood pressure and heart rate, we are doing less damage to our bodies, and thus, will look and feel better for longer.

Staying positive is very important. When we are thinking negative things, we look and act negative. We perceive life as being negative and act accordingly. Change your perception to the positive. Keep your posture straight and look people in the eye, smile. When you take on the posture of being positive, you will find it easier to be positive. Do not let the negative emotions take hold of you, avoid the stress that they cause on your body and change your outlook to a more positive one.

If you are a pessimist, you can break the habit. For each negative thought that you have, replace it with three positive ones. Pay attention to the little things that make you happy, stop rushing through your life. Avoid monotony, find new things to do every week or month and set small goals for yourself. Tackle that spare room you wanted to re-arrange. You will feel good as each one is accomplished.

Let go of any anger, regret or sorrow about the past. It is okay to say that we have made a mistake, acknowledge it, learn from it, and move on. Things happen in life that we have no control over, things that make us sad, hurt, or angry. We have no control over outside events but we can control how we react to them. If people in your life are, negative or seem to bring you down, distance yourself from them. You cannot choose what people around you say or do but you can control how you let it affect you.

Do not be afraid to cry when you need to. Holding back tears will hold back all the emotions, and you will carry that with you inside and it is not a good thing to do. Crying makes you feel better, it allows you to get out the pent up feelings and then you can deal with the grief and hurt instead of carrying it with you, where it will be another stressor on your body.

Laugh. Laughter is a good thing, as long as you are not laughing at the expense of another person. Laughter releases those endorphins that help keep your immune system and your heart healthy.

Enjoy the little things in life. Stop rushing through life, stop, and literally smell the roses. Take a walk in the park, on the beach. See a movie or go out to eat. Listen to the birds singing outside your window. Get a pet, take your dog for walks that benefit both of you or get a cat and spoil it. Petting a cat has been proven to help reduce stress and the cat will enjoy it too.

Lifestyle

We have all heard the phrase before; you are what you eat. However, it is very true. Our bodies must process and breakdown all that we put inside or ourselves in order to make it useful; the liver and kidneys filter out toxins. As we age, so do our organs and they may not work so well, especially if we have not been putting things that are good for us into them.

If you smoke, stop. Smoking has zero positive health benefits. To look younger, stop smoking, the sooner you stop smoking the better of a chance you have of reversing the damage that you have done. Not only does smoking increase your risk of cancer and does significant damage to your lungs, but also it affects your appearance, and none for the better. Smoking shrinks the blood vessels in your skin, reducing healthy blood flow so if you get a small cut it will take longer to heal with diminished blood flow. The collagen in your skin deteriorates; you lose the elastic nature of your skin. Your skin becomes dry and wrinkled. Your lips and teeth become stained from nicotine. Smoking adds age to your appearance, makes you look older than you really are.

Kick any drug habit that you have. Not only will drugs cause you numerous physical ailments, but also they affect how you look and how you feel. Illegal drugs will cause you to look older than you are and give you a sickly appearance. Take prescription medication only under a doctor's care and follow the directions for all over the counter medication. Taking more than you should for over the counter medication can damage your liver and kidneys, two vital organs. Read labels carefully and never take medication for something that you do not need.

Excessive drinking will not only affect your health but it will damage your skin as well and your state of mind. Drinking occasionally can actually benefit you. Wine has flavonoids in it and studies have proven that the occasional glass of red wine or wine can benefit your health. Excessive drinking does not benefit you. Not only will it have ill effects on your liver and kidneys; when you liver and kidneys are not working right, toxins build up in the body.

Get plenty of sleep. Lack of sleep can make you feel groggy and disconnected. Your memory will suffer and so will your response time to things. Your attention span will be shorter, your moods will be affected, and you will have mood swings. Lack of sleep can diminish the effectiveness of your immune system. Make sure you get plenty of rest. After a stressful day, try meditation. The breathing and peaceful nature of meditation will increase the oxygen flow into your body making you feel and look younger and better.

Stay active. You can do this by either exercise or by taking up a hobby, as long as you are active and staying busy. Start a garden, build a birdhouse, crochet, or knit, play music or sing, take up woodworking or even car restoration. Just stay active. When you have long bouts of inactivity, you start to feel stiffened up and lose your balance and are prone to injuries. Stay active to avoid this.

If you are overweight, lose the weight with a balanced diet and exercise plan. Avoid crash diets or fad diets. They work in the short term but are denying your body the nutrients and vitamins that it needs to work properly. Even if you just spent 10-15 minutes a day doing some sort of exercise, you will see and feel the benefits. Take walks, do yoga, water aerobics are a low impact exercise that is especially great for people who are older and just starting an exercise regimen.

A balanced and healthy diet is key to looking younger. Watch your fat and sodium intake. Add fiber to your diet. Use whole grain bread instead of white bread. Eat more fruits and vegetables. Not only do you get many vitamins from fruits and vegetables, but you get many other health benefits from the other things they provide such as: Phytochemicals that lower your risk of cancer and boost your cardiovascular system and act as anti-oxidants, organosulfur compounds that help your body fight off heart disease and stroke, carotenoids that help us fight off disease and reduce the risk of cancers, tannins that help us fight cancer and heart disease and lowers our risk of having a stroke.

Take vitamins and supplements. The most important ones to have in your diet are Vitamin A, Vitamin B, Vitamin C, Vitamin D, and Vitamin E. You can often find a daily supplement that contains all of these. Each of these serves a purpose in our bodies and when we lack one or all, we may start to look older and not feel as good.

Environment

What you surround yourself with is equally important as what you put inside of your body. External factors also take a toll on our looks and can age us prematurely. The things that we breathe, eat, drink, or touch can have a negative effect on our health and our looks. We do not have any control over our genetics but we can control our environment to some degree.

With the advance of science, the number of chemicals and chemical compounds are increasing. Smog, pollution from factories, commercial pesticides on the foods that we buy, pollution from cars, cigarette smoke, pesticides for home, cleaning supplies, even the artificial additives and preservatives in our foods can all have a negative effect.

As we age, our bodies will slowly begin to lose the ability to rid itself of the toxins that can cause damage to our organs. To look and feel, your best you need to really need to limit what you are exposing yourself too; limit the toxins that you take in.

Pollution, especially smog, has been linked to heart attacks, several chemicals used in industrial processing plants are carcinogens, industrial areas have higher instances of breast cancer, and certain cancers are more common among those who use certain pesticides in agricultural areas.

Smog in the cities is a mixture of chemicals, none of which will do you any good. Avoid being outside during rush hour. Pay attention to pollution alerts and avoid being outside during that time. Make sure that you get away from the smoggy areas to get fresh air if you live in the big cities. On your days off enjoy a walk someplace where the air is fresh. Go someplace off the beaten path and away from the traffic. The fresh air will do you good and keep your skin looking better.

Do not smoke and avoid your exposure to second hand smoke. We have already gone over the damage that smoking does to your body so we will not go back over that. However, the second hand smoke it just as dangerous to your skin and body. Keep your home a smoke free environment. Get a home air purifier with a HEPA filter and keep your filter clean. Keep your home environment as clean as possible to filter out the pollution in the air.

Limit your exposure to the sun, wear sunscreen if you are outside. Sun exposure is not only a major factor in skin cancer but it also dries out the skin, causes wrinkles and your skin will lose its elasticity. Wear a hat and sunscreen if you are outside. Do not use tanning salons; that is just exposing your skin to artificial UV rays and will damage your skin in the long run.

Limit the use of household chemicals and pesticides. Look for all natural cleaning products to use around the house. Use cleaners that use lemon and orange oils instead of harsh chemicals. Find organic ways to deal with any pests in the house instead of insecticides.

Commercial farms use pesticides to control bugs and plant diseases. Always wash the fruits and vegetables that you buy from the supermarket. As an alternative, you can look for foods labeled as pesticide free and all organic. Be wary of the artificial ingredients and preservatives in the foods that you buy. Limit your intake of processed food items and eat organic products. Start a garden and grow some of your own fruits and vegetables. They will taste better than food grown in a greenhouse. Gardening is also a good activity and a great hobby.

Just be aware that the things that we surround ourselves with can also prematurely age us. Limit the exposure and we retain that youthful look a lot longer. Read labels. Pay attention. Be more aware of what chemicals you are exposing yourself to either by air, touch or through eating and drinking.

Tips to Look Good – Quickly

We all want to be more attractive and make a great first impression. Being attractive is not just about looks, it is also about charisma. Our world is fast-paced; we want to stand out, both in the business world and in our personal life. As unfair as it is, first impressions count. We will help you make your first impression be a great one. We will also help you maintain your body image, your charisma and your attitude so that you continue to impress people and make a positive impression upon people.

Think of the politicians, the business leaders, and the celebrities that are just showstoppers. They have confidence, an allure and a magnetism to them that makes them a success that goes far beyond just their looks.

People who make a positive impression, the ones that have the magnetic personality and the charismatic personality all share some common traits. They are go-getters, they get the job done and often on their own initiative, they more dominant and less submissive. They make eye contact and enjoy interacting with people. They are expressive and their body language is open and inviting. Their posture is good and they lean in when listening instead of having a closed and uninviting body language. Their appearance is always attractive and appropriate for the occasion. They wear stylish clothes and accessories. They speak in a strong voice and speak clearly. They get things done, but do not rush. They have a positive outlook and demeanor and are always confident.

These are all traits that you too can have. There is no secret club to being more attractive and successful; it is all within your reach already. Do not waste time wishing you were one of those people that you admire, start being one of them. We will help you feel energized, attractive and you will learn how to be influential, charismatic, and even seductive. You will be more confident in both your business and your personal life. You will look and feel more positive and more attractive. You will be confident and people will notice you.

This goes beyond just a simple make over. We are not talking plastic surgery or expensive procedures. We are talking about the entire package. How you present yourself, tailoring your wardrobe for maximum impact, your way of interacting with others, even your attitude is important.

Here are some of the key areas that we will work on:

Body Language

- Posture

- Mannerisms

- Your Facial Expressions

- Personal Space

- Eye Contact

- Using Touch

Physical State

- Healthy Appearance

- Being in Shape

- Wear a Smile

Your Style and Manner of Dress

- What to Wear

- Find Your Style

- Accessorize yourself

Your Presence

- Pace your Movements and Speech

- Take Command of Your Area

- Eye Contact

Body Language Counts

Body language is vital. When somebody meets you for the first time, his or her first impression of you is of your appearance. You may hold all of the secrets to the world in your brain but if you are slouched against a wall and meet people with a limp handshake and no eye contact, it does not matter because they will already have formed an impression of you; a negative one.

Watch your posture; keep your posture balanced with your weight evenly distributed between both feet. Hold your back straight but naturally so, not rigid and keep your shoulders back and down. This will make you appear more assertive and an appearance of strength and vitality. Watch how you hold yourself when stressed, tension will make your shoulders bunch up and your body a tendency to lean or slouch. When feeling stressed, take several deep breathes and relax your shoulders as you breathe out. Do this five times and you will feel less stressed and more centered.

Keep your body language open. When your body language is open and relaxed it shows that you feel positive, makes you more approachable by others and shows that you have confidence. When you have closed body language, such as slouching, not making eye contact, keeping your arms across your chest you but up signs that you do not want to be approached and that you are uncomfortable, and lack confidence. Keep your hands in view; do not hide them in your pockets. When you keep your hands in view, people tend to view this as a trait of openness and honesty. When talking to another person, never stand directly opposite, as this is a challenging stance. Stand at a slight angle to them to appear more friendly and open.

Be aware of your expressions. Avoid passive aggressive non-verbal negative motions such as rolling your eyes or sighing deeply. When speaking to others, watch their body language as well as a cue to how the conversation is going so you can reply appropriately. When somebody has a downturned mouth, they are likely sad and approach them as such. Angry people often have a frown, furrowed brows, narrowed eyes, and tightened lips. Happy people will be smiling, their eyes will be open, and the smile is genuine and reaches both sides of the mouth. A person with a one-sided smile is often arrogant and mocking. A scared person tends to stare, their face is tense, their body is tense, and their breathing is often faster than normal.

Making eye contact is essential. When you make eye contact, you give an impression of sincerity, honesty, and confidence. Always make eye contact when communicating with people but do not hold eye contact for too long. Prolonged eye contact can be interpreted as a sign of aggression. While speaking to somebody, make frequent eye contact. If you do not make enough eye contact the person you are speaking to may think you are not interested, are not being sincere, lack confidence and when you do so you project feelings of shame, shyness, insecurity and even sadness. A person who makes frequent eye contact with you is usually feeling attracted to you, a genuine interest in the conversation, and a genuine interest in you.

Keep a smile on your face; make sure you do not smirk. A lopsided smile signals disinterest, lack of sincerity, arrogance and makes you appear to mocking that person or feeling superior. Keep a smile on your face and be sure to watch how you have your head. Be sure to nod to show interest and tilt your head towards the person speaking to you to show that you are listening. Keep your arms uncrossed. For the gentlemen, keep your legs uncrossed If you have the body language that you are interested, people will speak to you easily, if you frown or keep glancing away during a conversation, it shows that you have no interest in the conversation and the person will cut their conversation short and walk away.

Part of being confident and attractive is to be assertive and to be able to deal with people firmly but in a positive way. How are successful people able to surround themselves with positive people? They are not mind readers. They have simply learned to read body language of the people they deal with. They can read from the actions or expressions whether they are talking to somebody who might be lying, anxious, or uncomfortable with the conversation.

Here are some signs of anxiety that you can look for:

• They fidget and appear restless

• Often touching themselves, especially around the neck or face

• Often will rub their forehead

• Chain smoking, excessive drinking or even overindulging in food

Here are some signs exhibited by people who are being deceitful

• Fidget in place

• Often have their hand covering their mouth

• Will not make eye contact or keeps breaking eye contact

• Blinks rapidly

• Stiff posture

- Seems to be deliberately holding their face devoid of expression

How you present yourself makes a difference in how other people perceive you. These traits will allow you to appear more in control and attractive to others, you will feel and appear to be more confident, friendly, and approachable. So remember to keep yourself open and friendly in posture, do not hide your hands in your pockets, show that you are interested in the conversation and make eye contact.

The Attraction Factor

You are not only looking to get noticed in the business world, you are also looking to attract men or women for relationships. Once again, romantic attraction is not all about looks; it is about the entire package. Remember, that the majority of the first impression is the image that you project.

You can be the most attractive person in the room but if your body language is closed up, you will also be the loneliest person in the room. Attraction is not just about looks, it is also about the aura about you. Do you appear to be available and friendly? Do you come across as unfriendly and unapproachable? If you want to be approached, you must make yourself approachable by others.

If you slink into a room and find a corner to lean against or a chair in the back to hunker down at, expect to not get any notice from others. Make sure to circulate around the room during a party. Gestures and movement are eye catching and get you noticed, touching your hair, arms or hands will draw others eyes to you as they catch your motion. Dress to impress but stay tasteful in what you wear, especially for the females; revealing is good, revealing too much is not good. When approaching people at a party do not come up from behind them; that will catch them off guard. Always approach people from the side or from the front, coming up from behind is often seen as threatening as if you tried to throw them off guard. Wear the most important thing you own, your smile.

Watch other people's body language for signs that they may be interested. How do you know what to watch for?

Body language clues that females often use to express attraction and interest:

• Lowered eyes after making eye contact

• Tend to flutter their eyelashes more often

• Will tend to look back up quickly again through their eyelashes after lowering their glance – giving a coy look

• Glancing over their shoulder to make eye contact with you

• Smiles while talking or listening to you

• Touching her hair often, licking her lips or touching her face, chest or arms often

• Stand closer to you

Body language clues that men often use to express attraction and interest:

• Smiles when talking and listening

- Small adjustment motions such as playing with their tie, adjusting their tie or their cufflinks, fixing their hair.

- Tend to take up more space when talking to somebody they are interested in, stand with a wider stance, taking up more room.

- Stand with a wide stance, the straddle, standing with their hands on their hips, moving their jacket back, displaying their crotch area more this way.

It is important to not only watch your own body language, but you can get valuable clues from the other person's body language as well. When speaking to somebody you are interested in, be sure to engage in conversation, even if nervous. Do not simply nod or give yes or no answers. Attraction is also about having a connection to the other person so be sure to give them a sense of who you are through conversation. Just nodding and one-word answers do not project a very good image and makes it hard to get to know you. Small talk is not easy for everybody, yet the attractive people, the powerful people seem adept at it. Get yourself used to talking to people throughout the day. At the grocery store, ask how the checker's day is going or the gas station attendant, or the server when you go out to eat. Soon you will be more relaxed when making small talk, it never hurts to be nice to the people you deal with along the way either.

Make a Power Play

Attractive people have an animal magnetism about them, a powerful presence that is both alluring and powerful. You do not want to be the person always on the fringes, on the peripheral of the action. You want to have presence also. If you want to make an impression, to have that presence, you need to make a power play. Here are some tips to becoming a dominant person in a group, ways to appear more confident and powerful.

When you are watching press conferences or award ceremonies, do you see anybody slouching in their chair or while standing? No. Even if you are not tall, give the appearance of height by standing straight. This is the easiest way to appear to be in control and confident. Watch your posture always. Do not fold up into yourself. Power and confidence is shown by taking a powerful stance and your use of space. Do not sprawl across the people around you, but take up your space by placing your hands on your hips and keeping your feet apart. Ladies, stand with one leg slightly in front of the other one. When you see stars pose on the red carpet, do they stand with their arms at their sides, feet together and head down? No! They have their head high, one or both arms on their hip and one leg out. This dominant stance shows that you are confident, and confidence is alluring. It shows you are self-assured. Do not hide behind other people and peek around their shoulders. Find your own space and be noticed. People who stay willingly in the background are not perceived as being confident and powerful. Do not be afraid to stake out your territory in a group setting; do not let yourself be pushed into the fringe of the group.

Always have yourself in check when it comes to your emotions. Always stay calm and relaxed on the outside, show people that you have control of yourself and the situation at hand. There is nothing attractive about coming apart in the midst of a crisis. There is something attractive and powerful about the person who holds it together when everybody else falls apart. Learn to manage your stress when things get out of control. Keeping your posture straight and taking deep breaths will help you calm down.

Watch your manners when entering and leaving a room. Hold the door open for others and be the last to either enter or exit a room that way. How you treat others is also a factor for attraction. Self-centered people who leave a room and let the door slam in the face of the person right behind them are not attractive people. Good manners will get you noticed and remembered.

When meeting people give a firm handshake but do not make it a contest for who squeezes the hardest. It is not a competition. Give a firm grip and not a limp grip. For an extra power play, touch the arm or shoulder of the other party at the same time as you greet them and give a handshake.

Do not speak to quickly or too quietly. Power play talkers are the ones that tend to keep the conversation lively and ongoing, will lean towards the people they are talking to and will express themselves through gestures as they talk. Make eye contact as you talk but do not hold the eye contact for so long that it becomes a challenging gesture. When in a group, make eye contact with each person.

These are the power play moves for standing out in a group setting. Your goal is to be noticed and in a good way. Saying hello to a few people and then hiding in a corner will never get you the confidence that you are looking for. Practicing these power plays will make you more confident and hence, more attractive. Just do not give up or lose heart. It takes practice to go from being a wallflower to a power player.

Quick Tips for Style and Fashion

You want to look your best and feel your best to be the best! When you take care of yourself, it shows that you value yourself. You want to be radiant and beautiful from the inside out. You need to watch what you put into your body and how you take care of it. Being attractive does not come from a cream or a pill, it starts with you, and how you take care of your body. When your body feels good, it shows in your face and skin and that makes you look good.

Take care of your skin. Healthy, glowing skin is alluring. Get enough sleep. Drink plenty of water throughout the day, at least 6 glasses of filtered water, to keep your skin hydrated and supply. Manage your stress with meditation and breathing exercises. Limit your sun exposure, wear sunscreen to protect your skin when you go outside. Make sure you have plenty of fiber in your diet, such as whole grain bread, fruits, and vegetables. Fruits and vegetables are also rich in antioxidants that help ride the body of damaging free-radicals that will age your body. Make sure to get enough essential fatty acids that are good for your body and especially your skin. Essential fatty acids are found in whole grains, soy, nuts, salmon, fresh tuna, dark green leafy vegetables, and cold pressed oils such as flax, pumpkin, sunflower and sesame. Help your body stimulate digestion and help rid itself of toxins by drinking a glass of warm water when you wake up; you can also drink warm water with lemon or nettle tea. Reduce the amount of alcohol, sodium and caffeine that you intake; they dehydrate your body and skin. Stay away from the following foods: foods with trans fatty acids, fried foods, excessive dairy, and red meat.

Keep your hair neat and tidy. Men, if your hair is longer, just keep it maintained and not shaggy. Women, for an extra wow factor, wear your hair up. Keep your hair combed and in control, keeping it tied up or put up in the workplace is very professional looking. To keep your hair thick and shiny, consider taking prenatal vitamins.

Never underestimate the effect of scent. Never have body odor. Always keep your hygiene regime up. The perfume and fragrance market is as big as it is for a reason; people love to smell nice.

A soft and subtle scent will get you noticed more than having no scent at all. Having a bad smell will get you a seat by yourself! Do not spray perfume on heavily and never re-spray yourself while at your desk at work. That is inconsiderate of your co-workers. A good tip to help your fragrance last throughout the day is to spray just above your head so the fragrance settles onto your hair and clothes and as you move the scent will seem to refresh itself. You can also spray in front of you and then walk into the mist as well. That is a good way to refresh the scent at work, but make sure you do this in the restroom or outside and not at your desk. You do not need to purchase expensive perfumes to smell nice. You can use essential oils, and body sprays and even scented lotions and get the same effect for a lower price.

Make sure you have a winning smile. Brush your teeth twice a day and get your teeth cleaned every six months by a dentist. Coffee, tea, and nicotine will all stain your teeth.

Avoid expensive treatments by following these tips to having great teeth:

• Certain foods will actually help whiten your teeth while you eat by exfoliating teeth before the molecules that stain have time to attach to the tooth's surface. Add the following foods into your healthy diet: apples, celery, spinach, broccoli, lettuce and carrots

• If your teeth are yellowish do not use dark shades of lipstick or shiny glosses instead use matte lipsticks in nude or pink shades that have a blue undertone

• If your teeth are grayish, use nude or pink lipstick with a brown undertone

- Use skin bronzers to give your skin a healthy glow, this makes the whites of your eyes and your teeth look brighter

- Wear silver or sparkling jewelry that make your teeth sparkle instead of wearing gold

- Do not wear bright white, wear off-white or cream shades instead

Wardrobe Know How

Attractive people dress to feel and look attractive. You do not see celebrities wearing ill-fitting outfits or stained clothing. Go through your closet and clear it out. If you have any of the following, throw them away: clothing that is too small, worn out or faded clothing, stained clothing, clothing that is very outdated and clothing that does not flatter your body type. Make sure to have color in your wardrobe. Color brings energy and life into your clothing. Even if you are wearing white or black, choose accessories with color for maximum impact.

This section is for the men. To be attractive, you must always dress to be attractive. Dress to fit the occasion, always. Keep in mind that powerful and attractive people value themselves and their image greatly so you should too. Wear good quality clothing and ditch anything with stains or holes. Even when at the gym or making a fast grocery store run; you never know who you will run across and you want to always give a great impression. Dress to hide your problem areas and accentuate your positive traits.

Here are some style tips for the men:

Problem Area = Short/Thick Neck

What to Wear

- Low neck and V necks shirts

- Shirts with narrow collars

- Discreet slim ties

What to Avoid

- Polo shirts and turtle necks

- Wide ties with loud designs

Long/Skinny Neck

What to Wear

- Polo shirts, worn buttoned up

- A neatly trimmed beard

What to Avoid

- V-neck and open neck line shirts

- Narrow ties

- Shirts with long pointed collars

Broad Shoulders

What to Wear

- V-neck shirts

- Vertical stripes

- Tight tops

- Knitwear

- Raglan sleeves

What to Avoid

- Clothing with padded shoulders

- Horizontal stripes

- Knits with patterns

- Baggy and loose fitting tops

- Shirts with dropped shoulder seams

Short Legs

What to Wear

- Jackets that just cover the seat of you pants, no extra length

- Vertical patterns and stripes

- Pants that fit up higher on the waist

- Pinstripe suits

- Narrow ties

What to Avoid

- Turn ups

- Pants and jackets with contrasting colors

- Double breasted jackets

- Pleats on the waist

- Wide belts

Too Tall

What to Wear

- Long Line and double breasted jackets

- Trousers with wide belts

- Horizontal stripes on tops

- Checks or patterned pleats

- Trousers low on waist

What to Avoid

- High rise trousers

- Vertical patterns

- Thin ties

- Short jackets

- Narrow belts

- Single breasted jackets

Beer Belly

What to Wear

- Slightly loose but well fitted clothes

- Wide tie ending at top of belt

- Straight line trousers

- Vertical print/stripes

- Single breasted suits

What to Avoid

- Very loose tops and bottoms

- Tight tops

- Pleated trousers

- Double breasted suites

- Short and narrow ties

Clothing Guide tips for the Women:

Square Shoulders

What to Wear

- Scoop or crew neck shirts

- Three quarter sleeves

- Jackets in darker colors

- Single breasted jackets

- Thicker shoulder straps

What to Avoid

- Double breasted, boxy tops

- Shoulder seams that fall on shoulders

Flabby Arms

What to Wear

- Three quarter sleeves

- Floating cuffs

- Puff at shoulder seam

- Fluted sleeves

- Delicate bracelets

What to Avoid

- Cap sleeves

- Sleeveless shift dresses

- Chucky bangle bracelets

Short Legs

What to Wear

- Straight leg or slight bootleg cut pants

What to Avoid

- Tapered legs

- Large pleats

- Boxy skirts

Large Backside

What to Wear

- Side Fastening and slightly loose fitting pants

- Slim line jackets ending under your backside

- Flared or pencil skirt

- Fitted dresses but no shifts

What to Avoid

- High waist and tight pants

- Jackets ending just above or on you backside

- A-line and straight skirts

Small Bust

What to Wear

- High neck tops and sleeveless tops

- Halter neck

- Ruffled front tops

What to Avoid

- Scoop and V neck tops

- Low cut sweaters

Large bust

What to Wear

- Wrap tops, v necks, scoop neck shirts

- Tops that are tighter on the waist and looser around the top

- Fitted jackets, deep v, cut to the hip

- Wrap dresses, empire dresses, three quarter length sleeves

What to Avoid

- Turtle necks

- Boxy jackets

- Halter neck

Take Care of Your Skin

You want to make the very best impression that you can. You want to dress to impress and look impressive and youthful at the same time. Your skin is a vital piece of you that you want to take care of and nourish. The largest organ in the human body is the skin, so you want to take care of it because when you do not take proper care of your skin, you will look older than you really are and can have a sickly look. You want to be a power player, you want to be charismatic, attractive and make an impact. Your skin is made up of several aspects and the ones that need your attention the most are: collagen, elastin, fibroblast cells, and connective tissue. In order to properly take care of your skin you will need to include the following in your skin care regime: cleaning, toning, moisturizing, sun protection, skin treatments.

Make sure you drink six to eight glasses of water a day in order to keep your body flushed of toxins and to keep the skin hydrated. If you do not get enough water into your body, no amount of moisturizer will be able to protect your skin. Your skin has two layers, the epidermis, which is the outer layer and the dermis, the inner layer. The dermis is what gives your skin the elasticity and strength. When your skin is in poor condition, the dermis loses its elasticity; the skin will sag and wrinkle. Regular facials or even at home facial massages with pure oils such as olive or almond will help prevent that from happening.

It is important to clean your skin twice a day. Cleaning removes dirt and oils that build up on the surface of the skin and blocks pores. Blocked pores will cause blackhead and whiteheads to appear. If you have pimples, do not pop them! You can get a cream to dry out the pimple, and it will heal without the scab and scarring that popping a pimple will cause. To prevent the skin from drying out when washing it, use a gentle pH balanced soap or cream wash. Always remove your make up before going to bed using cold creams or a gentle make up remover, especially around the eyes and then wash your face with the gentle cleanser. Use an exfoliating wash or scrub once or twice a week to remove dead cells and help keep your skin looking radiant.

To help your skin retain that youthful glow and shine, after washing your face, use a toner about twice a month after washing your skin. Things like weather, pollution and harmful factors in the environment will make skin look dull, feel dry and impure. Using a toner twice a month will clean the oils and impurities trapped in your skin, giving you a rejuvenated look and feel to your skin. Skin toning lotions will help increase the blood supply to your skin, keeping it more elastic and healthy for longer than if you do not use toners.

Washing will remove oils from the surface of the skin, so it is important to use a moisturizer to replace these oils and give your skin a protective barrier. For problem skin, look for a non-pore blocking and water based creams. You can use a thicker cream for nighttime. Only you know what kind of skin you have and so choose your moisturizer based on what type of skin, there are endless kinds out there.

Protecting your skin from the sun is a must. Always wear sunscreen, even if you only use a moisturizer with a built in sunscreen or sunscreen on top of your normal moisturizer. Rays from the sun will cause wrinkles and premature aging as well as exposing you to skin cancer in the long term.

Skin treatments depend on what kind of skin problem that you are having. For large pores, you can find clay masks to help draw out the impurities or special creams to help reduce pore sizes. Both dry skin and oily skin have special creams as well as for diminishing skin or age spots on the face. There are treatment masks and creams for any skin problem. Do not be afraid to read the boxes, see what product is good for you. Department stores have extensive skin products by various companies and the clerks are always very knowledgeable; do not be afraid to ask for their recommendations and product samples.

Anti-Aging

Nobody wants to age but it happens to us all. Fortunately, there are steps we can take to prevent us from looking older prematurely and even looking youthful while we age. Taking care of your skin goes a long way towards keeping a youthful appearance.

Here are some of the key things to look for in a skin care product for anti-aging:

Anti-oxidants – these reduce the process of cell damage that results in discoloration and wrinkles

Look for products containing: green tea, grape seed, ascorbic acid, retinyl palmitate, ginko bilboa and Japanese alder

Anti-Enzymes – these maintain the elasticity and firmness of your skin

Look for products containing: echinacea, hydrocotyle, grape seed extract, flavonoids and green tea

Anti-Inflammatories - these reduce redness and puffiness of the skin

Look for products containing: licorice, green tea, cucumber, chamomile, sage, red clover, Canadian willow herb, sinanediol, avena sativa

Cellular Stimulants – these encourage healthy skin cells and stimulate cell growth

Look for products containing: vitamin a, Echinacea, ergothioneine, sage, red clover, wheatgerm extract, bioflavonoids, coralline officinalis

Emollients and Protectors – these protect the surface of the skin – avoid lanolin and mineral oil because they will block your pores causing more skin problems in the long run

Look for products containing: shea butter, algae extract, cyclomethicon, phospholipids, retinyl palmitate

Avoid products that contain the following harmful ingredients: propylene glycol, mineral oil, sodium lauryl sufate, and sodium laureth sulfate.

To keep your skin looking younger and healthier looking there are some things that you need to do, and avoid. Always use sunscreen or moisturizer with minimum spf 15 all year round. Get plenty of sleep and learn to relax and reduce stress that may cause you to not get enough sleep; try meditation or guided relaxation along with breathing exercises. Take care of your skin by keeping it clean, exfoliated and moisturized; night creams are especially important as you can hydrate your skin much better and can use a thicker cream. Use quality skin care products, read the labels, be aware of what you are putting on your skin. Reduce your alcohol intake and do not smoke. Stimulate circulation by massaging your face or having a facial massage done at the spa with a facial.

Your lifestyle affects you and your appearance just as much as what you put onto your skin. Watch what you eat. If you eat a diet full of high fat and high calorie food, you are depleting your body of nutrients and preventing your body of filtering out and eliminating toxins. Some lifestyle tips to consider are:

Have a good balanced diet with plenty of fresh and raw foods, especially vegetables and fruits

Eat a diet with plenty of fiber to keep your system regular and to help prevent toxins from building up; eat plenty of whole grain foods

Eat vegetables and fruits rich in anti-oxidants to help stay healthy and rid your body of free radicals

Exercise – keep in shape and both look and feel healthy.

Use probiotics to help keep your system regular

Learn to relax and shed stress from your life

Have good relationships – we all need people that are positive in our lives

Community support and involvement – be involved, helping out makes you feel good and valued

Quick Tips to Look Young

Nobody wants to go the party and dress older than they are or end up looking frumpy. You want to look attractive and look young. There is nothing worse than ending up with somebody assuming that you are years older than you really are upon meeting for the first time. Thankfully, it is very easy to avoid.

Look as natural as possible. Do not go with hairstyles that would stand up to a gale force wind; avoid stiff hairstyles. Go for a style that allows your hair to move as you move, even if you wear your hair up, avoid weighing it down with gels and sprays. Go for the natural look with your foundation and powder as well. Do not use so much foundation that it cakes and looks unnatural. Look for light coverage foundations or use a tinted moisturizer instead. Use a light liquid foundation or a mousse foundation to avoid having it cake.

Avoid having dark circles under your eyes; dark circles make you look like you are sick, not sleeping or that you lack vitality. Some people are born with dark circles under their eyes, for those that are genetically pre-disposed to having dark circles, get an under eye cream that targets the eye area and use a good concealer. Concealers with a yellow base are excellent for covering up dark circles. The rest of us will still get dark circles mostly from a poor diet, not enough sleep, or stress. Always drink plenty of water and get at least 15 minutes of exercise a day, even if just a brisk walk around the block once or twice. There are many creams to combat this problem but if you want a natural remedy, you can use potatoes. Grate a raw potato and fill a thin cloth, such as muslin or cheesecloth, with the grated potato and place over your closed eyes for 10-15 minutes. The starch in the potato will lighten the skin and you can use this home remedy every other day.

When your skin has a poor texture or excessive wrinkles it makes you look aged and unhealthy. You can use micro dermabrasion and minor surface peels. Never have any peels or procedures done at any spa or salon without have references and licenses checked. A good home remedy to prevent poor skin texture is to apply a light coating of almond oil at night to your slightly damp face.

A good home remedy, for the occasion pimple…a dab of toothpaste! A small dab of toothpaste before bed will help the inflammation go down.

Avoid using dark intense colors on your lips, use pinks or light reds or bronzes instead with some gloss on top to give your lips a youthful shine. Avoid the heavy-handed eyeliner and mascara look.

For a younger look, use browns or colors instead of blacks.

Yellow or stained teeth will age you quickly! Opt for whitening toothpaste and the at home whitening. For severely stained teeth, see your dentist for professional whitening treatments. Keep your nails trimmed and use either a clear coat or a light color on them. A good tip to prevent hangnails are to soak your nails in olive oil once a week, this will soften your cuticles and moisturizes your nails.

Use a bronzing lotion on your legs for some light color without the damage of tanning. Do not wear long flowing skirts that hide your figure. Use a more fitted skirt with a just under the knee or middle of the calf length to look younger and more feminine.

Wear shoes with some color and style to keep your look young and fresh. Accessorize, use scarves, earrings, rings, chains to add sizzle and color to your look.

Wear clothes that fit, nothing baggy or too large. Always have a well-fitting pair of jeans in your closet. A great pair of jeans paired with a classy top and some great shoes makes a great fast and easy way to go from your day to you evening without changing your whole look.

Makeup

Nobody is born with a naturally perfect face and makeup is a great way of hiding the imperfections and calling subtle attention to your highlights. The first step is always to wash your face and then moisturize. Wait 10 minutes after moisturizing before applying your makeup

Pick a foundation that blends with your natural skin tone, apply a light layer, and build up if you need extra coverage. If you are prone to oily skin, opt for an oil free and non-comdogenic foundation. Dry skin sufferers should use the liquid and cream foundation.

Use concealer to hide your problem spots. Yellow-based concealers will cover up bruises, eye circles, and mild red skin tones. A lavender based concealer will cancel our yellowish bruises, sallow skin, and dark spots on skin and very dark under eye circles. Green based concealers will cover up red spots and blotches and port wine stains.

Following up your foundation and concealer with a pressed or loose powder will set the foundation and make it last longer. It is also great for those prone to shiny skin, as it will absorb the oils that cause the shine.

Tame your eyebrows with tweezers or have them waxed at a salon. Avoid extreme eyebrow shapes that give you the "surprised look". For thin brows, fill in with an eyebrow pencil.

Your eye shadow should be three complementary colors. The lightest color opens your eyes and makes them brighten; you use this just under the eyebrow. The medium color will give depth to your eyes; use this color to cover your eyelid. The dark color will give depth and shape to your eyes; use this color to line along your upper lashes.

Eyeliner gives your eyes shape and definition. Highlight your eye color by using colored eyeliners. Avoid the heavy black eyeliners. Less is more when it comes to eyeliner, start with your upper lashes only, and if you need more color, line the lower lashes but only the outer 2/3 of the lashes.

If you have blue eyes, use shades of brown, camel, and taupe to make them stand out.

Use dark brown and charcoal color liner. If you have green eyes, use shades of plums, purples, browns, and brown-pink to make your eyes look greener. Use deep purples, dark browns, and charcoal for your eyeliner. If you have brown eyes, use shades of golden brown, slate blue, grey, and plum. Avoid light colored liners and use deep navy blue, cool dark browns, dark metal greys instead.

Use mascara to make your eyes look more detailed. Never overdo your mascara and go for colors instead of black. For think lashes, apply a second coat after the first coat has dried and use an eyelash comb to separate the lashes and remove clumps. If you have dark circles on your eyes, opt for black or brown-black mascara on the lower lashes instead of colored mascara.

The last thing to apply is your blush. Smile to find the plumpest part of your cheeks and apply blush to enhance your cheekbones. Use a light layer of rosy color blush and blend in. A flush on your cheeks will make you look radiant and healthy with a youthful glow to your face. Do not over apply or use a deep color blush.

When applying lipstick, opt for colors that suit your skin tone. If you have fair skin, you should wear berry, wine colored reds with a blue undertone, light to medium browns or beiges with a pink undertone. If you have olive skin, you should wear dark berry shads and deep brown reds. Avoid wearing pink if you have olive skin. If you have medium skin, you should wear deep pinks, deep reds, medium-brown and caramel shades with a pink undertone. If you have dark skin, you should wear reds with a blue undertone, wine reds and almost any shade of brown.

Personality Traits

Personality counts and it is something that you cannot simply fake. It is better to be yourself than to be caught trying to be somebody else. You have the traits within you already, and if one trait is stronger than the other, that is okay. Work on enhancing the traits that you have and the rest will fall into place. Nobody is perfect in every way, and nobody expects you to be either.

Always believe in yourself. Self-doubts are the enemy of what we are trying to accomplish. If you do not value yourself, nobody else will either. Train yourself to be positive, positive about yourself and about life. Never show yourself in a negative light. When you start to say a negative or if you are thinking in the negative, re-work it in your head before you say it. Turn that thought about not being skinny enough into a thought about how much you value your health and that you are happy that you are working on your health. Never think you cannot do something or express that you are not good enough. You are good enough if you think you are.

Do self-affirmations in the morning. Every morning when you wake up, say one thing about yourself that you love. At the end of the day, say one thing or achievement that you accomplished that day.

Set goals. When you set a series of small goals, they seem so be much more attainable than one vague far-reaching goal. As you reach each goal, rejoice in the fact that you met it and accomplished it. It will make you feel successful and like you are making progress. It will help keep your outlook positive, and your goals focused. It feels good to be able to cross a goal off your list as you finish it. Keep adding new goals and stay energetic.

Take 20 minutes out of the day to visualize what you want, what you goals are. See it in your mind, as you reach and finish each goal. Use meditation music to enhance this. Visualizing your goals in this manner will keep you energized as you see the success daily in your mind. This allows you to expect success and be more confident. Confidence is a power trait.

Do not take everything personally. If somebody snaps at you or is rude, do not assume it has anything to do with you because 99% of the time, it has nothing to do with you. Do not let somebody's bad day become your bad day. Remember that when things get bad, it could always be worse and indeed many people do have it worse than you do. Take stock of what you have and appreciate that. Always be polite and keep a smile on your face.

Before going into a meeting, or a sales pitch, do your research. Get to know what their background is, their interest, and their motivations, this is especially important in the business world. If you make the effort, they will notice and be impressed.

Play to the ego of the other party. Make them feel valued and important and they will remember that you did so. Do not go over the top so it feels faked. So be genuine, and be positive. Compliment their looks, the service at the company they work for or their work personally. Listen to what they say when they talk and ask questions or comment on what they say with something more than a yes or no response. Make them feel important that you are listening and caring about what they have to say. Even with small talk, keep it positive and upbeat! Do not complain and do not go into anything negative.

Know how to work the room in a group setting. When you enter, stop, and give the room a scan. Take note of where the other key people are. People will also notice the pause you gave as you entered the room, so keep your posture straight and confident. When talking, never turn you back to anybody. Always keep at a slight angle when speaking to them but keep them in view. When speaking, make sure your speech paced moderately, and take pauses to let what you say sink in. Do not prolong the pause, just a second or two is fine. This will also help you to not rush your words or speak too fast. When you take a pause, make sure to make eye contact with the person or the people listening to you, and then continue. Make them feel like you are truly speaking to them. People like people who make them feel important.

Professional Success

When it comes to your business success, nobody wants to be the person who just makes the goals or does the bare minimum, never advancing in the company. You want to be the person that does not ask for a promotion, you want to be the person that management wants to promote, without you asking.

Success does not rely on your looks alone. You want to make an impact and be a power player at work. That means to dress for success and take care of yourself but it also means that you have that can-do attitude. Nobody gets ahead at work by keeping his or her head down and staying quiet. Find your voice. Do not let a lack of confidence keep you from reaching your potential.

There are some very simple things that you can do to broaden your horizon and help to both appear and be smarter. Always speak clearly, do not mumble. If you do not have an answer, instead of a mumbled excuse or attempt to explain, just clearly state that you do not know. You appear a lot smarter to others when you admit that you do not know the answer than when you get caught trying to fake an answer. Avoid slang terms and words and do not swear. If somebody uses a word you do not understand, ask him or her, what it means rather than answer the question or comment on his or her statement; a poor attempt at guessing the meaning is an obvious thing. In addition, if you ask for a meaning, it shows that you are both willing to learn new things and able to admit when you do not know something.

Watch your manners. Good manners will get you noticed in a good way, so always be polite. Power players care about the people around them and it shows. Do not hang back and wait for people to approach you; introduce yourself to people you do not know. Make small talk and get to know them a little bit. If you see somebody without a drink, offer to get them one; manners, remember. Keep it positive! No complaining, stay upbeat and have a positive tone. Keep a smile on your face, hand out compliments, and if a conversation turns negative, excuse yourself and walk away. Do not engage in gossip.

Having trouble remembering names of the people you met?

In your spare time, practice ways to boost your brainpower. Learn one new word a day and try to use it at least once that day. Read book; find an author that interests you and read. Look up words you do not understand. This will help expand your vocabulary and keep your brain active. Hone your weak areas with classes and audio courses. There are many audio books and online lectures or classes to help you with areas you need help on. This can be public speaking, selling techniques or even learning computer programs such as Excel, PowerPoint, and Word.

When giving a presentation, combine all of these. Be engaging, tell a story, involve the audience, use humor. Do not make it a presentation about you; make it about "we", as if they and you are a team. Be prepared; know your audience. Find out who they are and what they are about and incorporate that in the presentation. Greet them warmly at the beginning and thank them for their time at the end. Have your presentation goals clear and easy to understand and have a structured presentation. Give them something to relate to such as case studies and visual aids like diagrams, photos, and charts.

If you are giving a meeting, learn to make a meeting a power meeting. Make it comfortable to the guests and to yourself. Use round tables to promote harmony and make it easier for all to be involved. Always offer a beverage, even if only cold bottled water and make sure the seating is comfortable. Take command of the meeting by introducing yourself and the other attendees and clearly state what the meeting is about and what their involvement is. Nobody likes to be part of a meeting and not know why he or she is there.

Energize Your Body

Your health is vital. You can be the most attractive person in the room but if you are wheezing with each breath or coughing every 5 minutes, it is not very attractive. You want to be attractive from the inside out. Your health starts with you; nobody else can get you fit and healthy.

Our environment can be damaging. Limit your use of cleaning chemicals and pesticides in favor of organic and all natural solutions. Help purify your air at home with air purifiers with HEPA filters. Add plants to your home for a touch of life and they help clean the air; plants such as spider plants, heartleaf philodendron and the peace lily.

Remember when your mom used to tell you to not sit so close to the TV because it was bad for you. She was right. Electro-magnetic fields produced by electricity and electrical appliances such as TV's and computers can cause insomnia, high blood pressure, and anxiety. Do not keep them near your bed and limit the amount of time you spent parked in front of them.

Have a peaceful spot to de-stress. Use flowers or plants to create an inviting home and they produce a better smell than any scent in a can. Have a spot where you can mediate, or reflect on the day and your goals. Install a birdbath in your yard or a bird feeder and watch the birds. Get a pet and pamper them, pets are great for stress relief.

Get fit. If you cannot afford a gym membership that does not mean all is lost. Join a community pool. Take a jog or even a brisk walk around your local park or your block. Buy home gym equipment for your house, there are stores out there that sell used equipment. Many communities offer classes such as yoga or aerobics for a small fee. The important thing is to get your heart rate up for 15 minutes a day to start getting healthy. Bring a pair of walking shoes to work and take a 15-minute walk at lunchtime even. Get your co-workers involved even.

Watch your diet. You are what you eat. The recipe for losing weight is simple, burn more than you intake. Do not starve yourself. You can eat healthy, nutritious, and filling foods and be satisfied.

Pass up the junk food and packaged snacks in favor of raw fruits and vegetables. Smoothies are a great way to get your fruit intake. Pass up the fast food and opt for a large smoothie for a meal or a small one for a snack. A good diet has the following heath improvements: lowers blood pressure, lowers cholesterol, improved insulin resistance, improved skin tone, improved weight and body tone, improve your immune system.

Avoid red meats, full-fat dairy, fried foods, Trans fats, excessive caffeine, and alcohol. Add whole grains and brown rice into your diet to get the complex carbs that are good for your health. Eat fruits and vegetables, but not the canned kind. Canned fruit is full of high fructose corn syrup. Eat as much organic and fresh food as possible to limit your intake of artificial ingredients and preservatives.

Sex Appeal

Being attractive is not just about looking good. It is about your personality, your charisma, your mind, and your body language. You need to be able to get their interest and seal the deal with who you are as well.

Banish your viewpoint of yourself being unlucky in love or as being shy or fumbling. Do not visualize the negative or it becomes true. You must think of yourself as being sexy and attractive in order for other to think of you as attractive. Start with positive affirmations, what do you like about yourself. What are you best features. Enjoy watching yourself walk in the mirror or talk. Fall in love with yourself. Visualization is a powerful tool so daily, find a quiet spot, and close your eyes. Imagine yourself as walking into a room and being confident, and looking and feeling great.

When you are interested in somebody, play it coy. Do not come on so strong that you appear desperate. Be relaxed, if you get nervous or anxious simply find a quiet spot, and take several deep breaths and do your positive affirmations. Be natural and relaxed and be teasing. Teasing perks interest and gives you that allure.

Manners count, nothing sexier than having somebody you are interested in anticipating your needs and being polite. For quieter settings, make sure to set the mood. Go someplace comfortable to you so that you are relaxed and more at ease but make sure it appeals to his or her interest as well. Do not plan a hike and a picnic for somebody who does not enjoy being outdoors.

Mix things up a little. Do not let things get stale by going to the same places and doing the same things. Find new places to explore together. Find things to do that appeal to you and him or her as well. Appeal to his or her interests, even if you may not be super keen on it but they will appreciate that you are doing things for them. That makes you more charming, sexier, and more appealing just for that.

You do not get what you want by hinting at it. Early on, being coy and teasing is a way to see if the other person is interested but it is not enough. If you prolong the tease factor, they may think that you are not serious and they will lose interest.

Be bold and go for what you want, have a hint of arrogance and a whole lot of confidence. Even if you are in a long-term relationship, never let the attraction die or peter out. Tell them you love them and tell them why. Compliments are never a bad idea and you can never give too many.

Add some spice to your relationship. Take things out of the bedroom and into another room for a change. Learn to give erotic or tantric massages. Have a surprise underneath your clothing. Buy some new lingerie or silk boxers and let them notice as you change after work or before bed. You can also tell them that you bought something new and sexy just for them but do not let them see it until bedtime. Take a local vacation; take the fun to a hotel room for a night, order breakfast in bed for a change. Keep the sex appeal fresh and fun in your long-term relationship. Try new things together and never let the romance die.

Express what you want. Know what you want and go after it, confidence is sexy and when you know that you have what they want, you feel sexy. Always speak up in bed and be positive. Keep a sense of adventure and fun in the bedroom; laughter is sexy and fun is alluring. Tell them what you like, and what you do not like. Do not let them discover what you do not like on their own and then reproach them for trying or doing it. That will deflate his or her ego and put a damper on the romance. Make sure to tell them what they do right, appeal to their ego and their sense of sexiness. Talk about what you would like to try or what you would like to try more of also.

Turn up the heat on the sex appeal. Tell them what you would like to do to them, make it smoldering.

Keep the heat smoldering by adding anticipation to what you would like to do when they get home. Leave a sexy voicemail on his or her cell phone, never the office phone! Give them something to look forward to.

Watch Out for Stress

Reduce your stress level by setting priorities, organizing, and setting attainable goals. Disorganization and feeling that you never make any progress is a huge cause of stress. Help eliminate this stress and make things easier by following a few simple hints and tricks.

Set a series of small specific goals to reach each day, each week, and each month. Write them down and cross them off as you reach each one. That gives you a feeling of getting things done, and indeed, you are. Do not make your goals vague, make them specific, like a to-do-list for each day.

Keep motivated and that will keep you productive. Visualize how you will feel when you goal is reached and how it will make you feel. This is your life and only you can be a success or failure, do not try to find blame with others for your mistakes. Take responsibility and learn from it.

Keep your life organized. Do not clutter and do not get overwhelmed. Keep your files and things that you need at work where you can reach them easily and have a system. At home, do the same thing. Avoid the temptation to dump everything on the dining room table to deal with later. Have a goal list for work and for home. Keep a calendar and write your business and personal things to do on them. Invest in a day planner or use an app on your phone to help you organize and set reminders to get things done.

Do not let deadlines sneak up on you so that you feel frantic and might make a mistake to finish it correctly. Use the A, B, and C method of priority for your work. A is the things that must be done today, B is the things that are urgent but can wait until tomorrow, C is the things that can wait at least 72 hours. Go through each stack daily because things from the C stack need moved to the B stack and so on.

Do not let interruptions stress you unnecessarily. When you have an interruption, close what you are doing on your desk to avoid getting papers shuffled. If the interruption involves something that you can complete in just a few minutes, go ahead and complete it to get it out of the way rather than letting it stack up.

Do not let your desk bog down with work. Things that you can get done quickly and out of the way, take care of them.

Do not let your stress build up at work. Take a walk outside for a few minutes. When you cannot step outside at your office, close your eyes, and take several deep breaths and then exhale slowly. This is a great way to get a quick burst of energy and to calm down. Never lose your cool at work or at home.

Learn to problem solve like a pro and avoid the stress that comes with major problems. When a problem happens, accept it. Take a realistic view of what the situation is and how you should best handle it. Research the problem and never be afraid to ask for help. Brainstorm with others and do not stress out over probabilities. Do not waste time coming up with too many solutions, the problem will be getting worse and your stress and anxiety level will just increase. Apply solutions as you come up with them, and learn from your setbacks. Do not despair or throw blame; stay positive and avoid negatives.

Be Positive

Always keep your life/work balance even. Learn to promote the positives in your life to make yourself feel good and look good.

Get your rest. Getting plenty of sleep has many benefits, such as:

- Restores our body and mind – allows us to relax and recharge. When we do not get enough sleep, our bodies show it.

- Has a calming effect – our minds go from feeling stressed to feeling more peaceful

- Improves our immune system

- Increases concentration – when you are well rested you are less likely to make mistakes

Work out the tension of the day by having a massage. Massage has the following benefits:

- Benefits the muscular system by relaxing and stimulating muscles, relieves soreness, tension, stiffness and spasm

- Benefits the circulatory system by decreasing blood pressure, improving oxygen and nutrient supply to cells

- Benefits the skeletal system by relieving stiff joints and improving posture and body alignment

- Benefits the nervous system by relaxing muscle tension that will in turn reduce your heart rate, blood pressure and circulation and can help with insomnia by giving you a sense of deep relaxation

- Get a mood boost by getting a massage. Feel your tension and aches melt away

When stress starts to take a toll, use breathing techniques to blow stress away. Stress and anxiety can cause us to breathe faster and that raises our heart rate, blood pressure, and our muscle tension increases.

Anxiety causes shallow and rapid breathing and a decrease in the oxygen in our blood. Increase the oxygen by making your breathing more efficient, and hence calming. Take a few deep breaths using your diaphragm, this is also called abdominal breathing and it is very effective to make you feel relaxed, energized and ready to tackle whatever comes your way. Take a deep breath in and exhale though your mouth then take another slow breath in and hold it for a count of 5 if you are able and then exhale through your mouth slowly, for a count of 8. Do this 5 times twice a day or whenever you are feeling stressed.

Follow your dreams, no matter how big or how small. To be positive, you need to have positive things in your life and doing something that you are passionate about it a great way to promote a sense of wellbeing and joy. Find a hobby, a cause to champion, food, music, art, etc. Teach what you know to others; find joy in their joy about something that you love. Enthusiasm is contagious so when you are passionate about something, it shows and will add to your charisma and appeal.

Last but not least is pleasure and sex. Other than the obvious, there are many benefits to sex: it burns calories; it increases our blood flow, reduces stress, and can relieve pain. Oh yes, pain relief! Sex releases endorphins that act as pain relievers. A healthy sex life helps you feel young. We have a hormone that is released upon arousal that contributes to cardiovascular health, functions as an anti-depressant, improves cognition, promotes bone growth and maintains and repairs tissues.

Sex and intimacy is a huge boost to our body and our mind. Touch is a powerful tool. Erotic massage and sex makes us feel sensual and sexy and when we feel sexy we are sexy. It improves our self-esteem and our mood levels.

Doing things that bring about a positive feeling, they will help you stay positive. Do not let the world swallow you up in stress. Know what you like and take time to enjoy it and de-stress. Life is full of positive things to do, never pass up an opportunity.

Energize Your Mind

Keep your mind positive, keep your mind active and your actions will follow. Remember, it is not just about looks, it is about the whole package.

Give your brain food; learn about new things, explore personal growth books or audio books, learn a new language or tighten up skills that you need to work on. You can never learn too much.

Stay away from negative influences. Balance out the news, which is never full of good news, with a sitcom or another favorite show. Limit your interaction with negative people. If somebody in your life is draining you of your energy and vitality, it will show, and you will begin to be just as negative as they are. Everybody is allowed a bad day, just do not let it become an eternal bad day. Spend more time with positive people and interact with them. Hone your social skills by talking to friends of friends. Listen to what others are saying, do not just nod or talk over them.

Enrich your world by learning new things and going to new places. Listen to uplifting music that has a beat and energizes you. Music is something our moods respond to quickly. Try new activities and take chances! Be daring and feel alive. Do not be trapped by fear of failure.

Do not let failure get you down. Power play people do not see failure as a reason to quit; they see it as a challenge to try harder! They learn from the errors and try again. Be positive about what the goal is and that even if this time you do not succeed, be assured that you will eventually, because you will not give up. Do not let the negative thoughts of others get in the way of your own goals.

Exercise the body and it exercises the mind. Exercise gives you stamina and can also release those feel good endorphins. When you look good, you feel good and a brisk walk can be a great pick me up on a bad day.

Bring light and happiness into your environment. At work, do not engage in the office gossip or complain just because the others are. Power players do not engage in negative behaviors and it is never attractive to listen to somebody whine about something that they have the power to change. Take a walk at lunch to get away. Eat outside to enjoy the fresh air rather than the break room where the gossip is. Remember; limit the negative influences in your life to be more positive. Put up pictures of your loved ones, a pet or even a peaceful vacation picture or scene. Keep a flower in a vase on your desk to smell for a quick perk up of mood. At home, have bright and airy colors in your house and open the curtains to let the sunlight shine into your house.

Recognize that the mistakes of your past are just that, in your past. Your background does not matter and it does not limit your potential. Same with anybody else though, never judge them by their past either. Positive, remember!

Keep your brain active. Work on a jigsaw puzzle at home or do the crossword while having your morning coffee. An active brain helps you feel energized and young. Indeed keeping your brain active and engaged can help ward off dementia as we age.

Always keep working on your social skills. The best way to get attention is to give attention. People love to have somebody pay attention to them and they remember when somebody does. Always be respectful and appreciate what they are saying. Remember, we all have opinions and yours may not always be right. Never start an argument. Give your opinion and if somebody disagrees, it is okay to debate it, but keep it friendly and agree to disagree. Ask what his or her interests are and try to find common ground. Keep conversations light and friendly. Positive interaction with other people is a huge stress reliever and mood booster as well as building confidence.

Conclusion

Only you can bring yourself from a background player into a power player. You want to look and feel young and attractive. You want the success that comes with being a power player.

Now you know that it is way more than looks. It is a whole lifestyle change but one that you can easily do and maintain. The key is to always believe in yourself and be confident. Being attractive means that you not only have the looks, but the charms and the know how to be a power player and get what you want out of life. Be charismatic, have allure, and have fun.

Above all, never ever let things get you down. Nothing is more repulsive than a frown or a negative attitude.